Embark On Your Journey

MINDFUL PRACTICE

A Beginner's Guide To Vibrant Living

MARY HIGGS

Copyright © 2023 by – Mary Higgs – All Rights Reserved.

It is not legal to reproduce, duplicate, or transmit any part of this document in either electronic means or printed format. Recording of this publication is strictly prohibited.

Disclaimer

The suggestions and practices in this book are not intended to diagnose or treat any medical condition, nor is any part of this book intended to serve as medical advice. Please consult a licensed healthcare provider regarding any medical questions or treatments. The author recommends common sense when contemplating the practices described in this work.

Praise for *Mindful Practice*

"Mary Higgs shares her story of trauma, recovery, and self-reflection and distills into a hopeful set of insights and practices that can help everyone on their healing path."

—Matthew Sanford, author of *Waking: A Memoir of Trauma and Transcendence*, and founder of Mind Body Solutions

"Mary Higgs has written a beautiful and compelling book about yoga and her journey with spinal cord injury. As a Yoga for Everyone advocate, this book is essential to understand what it means to jump into our self-awareness fully. The practices Mary Higgs offers us are contemplative, honest and accessible to everyone. It is an interactive road map to connecting your body, mind, and soul. Thank you for this work!"

—Dianne Bondy, author of *Yoga for Everyone* and co-author of *Yoga Where You Are: Customize Your Practice for Your Body and Your Life*

"*Mindful Practice: A Beginner's Guide to Vibrant Living* gifts the reader with simple, accessible tools to face life's challenges. Each beautifully written chapter, full of insight and hope, is an invitation to experience ease, soothing mindfulness and movement practices that encourage self-acceptance."

—Jennifer Kreatsoulas, PhD, C-IAYT, author of *The Courageous Path to Healing*

"*Mindful Practice* offers readers of all walks of life a powerful opportunity to infuse their life with an increased sense of intentionality, purpose and meaning. Mary's teachings, stories and prompts are insightful, engaging, and accessible. Mary's deep commitment to sharing these stories, practices and teachings is evident. I have no doubt readers will feel supported, inspired, and moved by *Mindful Practice* and what it unlocks in their own life."

—Melanie Klein, co-editor of *Yoga & Body Image: 25 Personal Stories About Beauty, Bravery & Loving Your Beauty,* and *Embodied Resilience: 30 Mindful Essays about Finding Empowerment After Addiction, Trauma, Grief, and Loss*

"*Mindful Practice: A Beginner's Guide to Vibrant Living* offers a practical and accessible path for anyone who is consciously exploring their spirituality. In this practical guide, Mary Higgs offers a combination of personal stories, meditations, physical practices, and inspiration, which add up to a complete and comprehensive guidebook for anyone who is lost in the thicket of their lives and desperately trying to find a way out into the open. Of course, the answer is always to turn within, and Higgs prompts us to do that over and over again. Instead of losing hope and being discouraged by life's thorns, she encourages us to look for the occasional blossoms and the open sky."

—Jivana Heyman, director of Accessible Yoga and Accessible Yoga School, and author of *Accessible Yoga: Poses and Practices for Every Body*, and *Yoga Revolution: Building a Practice of Courage and Compassion*

"Those of us who've spent a lot of time browsing the self-help sections of our favorite bookstores know that there are a whole lot of authors claiming to know the secret to happiness. We also likely know that the suggestions in these books are often overwhelming, confusing, or only applicable to folks with disposable incomes. Take heart, friends! Mary Higgs' *Mindful Practice* is not that! Mary's work is rooted in her lived experience and shared in a way that's accessible, simple, and inspiring. She knows her stuff, but she's never dogmatic; she guides you through and encourages you to make mindful practice your own. She never leaves you hanging but doesn't 'tell you what to do' either. Instead, she offers brilliant tools to empower you to connect with your own inner wisdom. And that is life changing. Whether you're a seasoned yoga practitioner or have never practiced a pose in your life, you'll feel seen, supported, and empowered by the practical magic within these pages."

—Kat Heagberg Rebar, author of *Yoga Inversions* and co-author of *Yoga Where You Are*.

"Mary poignantly wears her own healing journey with well thought out and accessible yogi tools with which to anchor ourselves, guiding us on a path toward clearer self-awareness and sense of agency. This is a beautiful book that holds many seeds of wisdom one can plant and continue to nourish over and over again."

—Sarit Z Rogers, ERYT, SEP

"*Mindful Practice: A Beginner's Guide to Vibrant Living* is a unique, very accessible guide to gentle self-inquiry, personal awareness, and self-love. Mary openly shares her personal journey and the tools she discovered along her path of navigating her life. The beautiful method she has created guides and encourages you to wrap your arms around yourself and give yourself a hug, whether you are new to mindfulness or are further along your wellness journey. As a lifelong yogi, I have read and studied countless books and practices to enhance my quality of life through everyday joys and challenges, including a diagnosis in 1999 of Multiple Sclerosis, a debilitating neurological condition that has no cure. Mary's 5-step exploration method has given me a fresh, compassionate way to view myself and my circumstances. I am excited to include this book in my daily practice; it will never gather dust on my shelf."

—Cherie Hotchkiss, ERYT, YACEP, YourOwnGentleApproach.com

"There is sweetness and encouragement in Mary's writings. Her experiences as a person with a disability are reflected in loving suggestions for an accessible and beginner-friendly Yoga practice. Practicality aside, Mary's journal prompts offer a fun and delightful invitation in the spirit of Julia Cameron's *The Artist's Way*."

—ML Maitreyi, founder and director of Accessible Yoga Sacramento/Tahoe

Table of Contents

Dedication	i
Acknowledgments	ii
About the Author	iv
Introduction	5
Getting Started	8
5-Step Exploration Method	10
Mindful Practice	12
How to Use Mantras	14
Section One: *Relax*	16
Chapter 1 Mantra: I am strong.	16
Chapter 2 Mantra: Relax, the world is working in my favor.	20
Chapter 3 Mantra: Follow higher self.	23
Chapter 4 Mantra: I am enough.	26
Chapter 5 Mantra: Relax and trust.	30
Section Two: *Listen*	34
Chapter 6 Mantra: I'll be Ok - no matter what.	34
Chapter 7 Mantra: I am thriving. I am playful.	37
Chapter 8 Mantra: Trust yourself.	40
Chapter 9 Mantra: I am grateful to be alive.	42
Chapter 10 Mantra: Listen with curiosity.	45
Section Three: *Feel*	49
Chapter 11 Mantra: I forgive those who have harmed me in my past and peacefully detach from them.	49
Chapter 12 Mantra: My body is alive; I feel mind, body, spirit.	52
Chapter 13 Mantra: Just be you.	56
Chapter 14 Mantra: Feel, restore, keep hope alive.	59
Chapter 15 Mantra: My heart is open.	62
Section Four: *Embrace*	67
Chapter 16 Mantra: I acknowledge my self-worth; my confidence is soaring. My life is just beginning.	67

Chapter 17 Mantra: I am powerful. 69
Chapter 18 Mantra: I am open to new experiences. 72
Chapter 19 Mantra: Center. Breathe. 75
Chapter 20 Mantra: I clearly see blessings all around me. ... 78
Section Five: *Accept* 82
Chapter 21 Mantra: Keep it simple. 82
Chapter 22 Mantra: Make friends with life. 85
Chapter 23 Mantra: I am here to flourish. I am blessed. 88
Chapter 24 Mantra: Dive into what scares you. 91
Chapter 25 Mantra: Accept who you are. 94
Afterword 97

Dedication

For my wonderful, beloved Husband, my best friend, my partner, and my greatest champion; thank you for walking every step in this journey with me.

For my amazing Mother, who deeply supported and encouraged every step of my healing journey. Even though she is no longer with us, her presence lives on every page. With love and heartfelt gratitude, thank you for everything, Momma. I miss you dearly every day.

Acknowledgments

Every mindfulness journey is different. As an online academic and a former journalist, community health educator and newspaper editor, I began my mindfulness path with many questions.

Am I doing this right? Should I be feeling overwhelmed? Is it normal to compare myself to lifelong mindfulness practitioners? When will I become an expert? What if my experience feels differently than the experiences described by my mentors, guides, or teachers?

As most teachers (myself included) well know, asking questions is the first step to learning. And there's more than one path to vibrant living and self-acceptance. One person, one guide or one expert cannot answer everything for you. They can provide guidance for progression. But in the end, our growth is not determined by someone else. We each have the ability within us to light our own path. The assignment, in my view, is to develop our own set of tools to open ourselves up to what blinds us.

I've been fortunate to work with many wonderful mentors and yoga teachers. They not only opened my world on many levels, but they provide solace and substance on my still-continuing path. While this is not an exhaustive list, I want to acknowledge those who made a difference in my life.

Thank you so much Melanie Klein, Matthew Sanford and Mind Body Solutions, Jivana Heyman, ML Maitreyi and the Accessible Yoga community, Jessa Baxter Peterson and Manhattan area yogis,

Alexandria Crow, Dianne Bondy and Amber Karnes, Jennifer Kreatsoulas, Cherie Hotchkiss, Kat Rebar, and Sarit Rogers. I deeply appreciate your support and kindness. You have been a beacon of hope on my journey. You helped me move forward despite fear. I'm grateful for our connection. Thank you.

Working with excellent guides and teachers has made a difference in my life. But in my case, learning to sit with questions and uncomfortable feelings continues to be my journey. I'm grateful I've found a practice that provides space for messiness. That is, my journey has taught me to embrace and accept the uncomfortable feelings that sometimes stopped me in my path. This work never ends. For me, I will always come to this work as a beginner. I start fresh every day.

My hope for this book is to encourage you dear reader to forge your own path. Use the tools in this book as fuel to step into your path without fear.

While no journey is without darkness, I hope this book provides the beginner with useful tools and courage. Taking the first step is scary. Believe me I know. But the answers are within you. You can live a more vibrant life. Trusting yourself is the first step.

About the Author

Mary Higgs, MA, is a respected writer, online educator, speaker, and empowerment coach. She has an extensive history as an active disability advocate working with organizations such as the Yoga & Body Image Coalition and Accessible Yoga. Developing a passion for mindfulness and becoming an Adaptive and Accessible Yoga Teacher transformed Mary's life in unexpected and profound ways. She loves sharing her message that transformation comes from within and that yoga and mindful practice is for everyone. As a Registered Yoga Teacher (RYT 200), Opening Yoga Instructor (OYI), and certified Yoga for All and Accessible Yoga Teacher, Mary teaches people to explore and trust their inner wisdom so they can live more authentically and fully. You can read about Mary's work in her chapter, "Coming Home to Adaptive Yoga" in the book, *Embodied Resilience Through Yoga: 30 Mindful Essays About Finding Empowerment After Addiction, Trauma, Grief, and Loss*. Mary's work has also been featured in Yoga International, Omstars, Devata Active, Yoga & Body Image Coalition, and Mind Body Solutions. Visit her online on Instagram @mary_yogiable and her website: YogiAble.com

Introduction

Each person has that golden nugget inside of them—a unique truth that leads to enlightenment and personal growth. I stumbled into my path after surviving a car accident when I was 19 years old. In simple terms, I went from being an extroverted athlete deeply invested in dance, sports, and cheerleading to learning to live with the physical and emotional trauma of a spine injury that left me with partial paralysis and limited mobility. I had no clue how to proceed with my life. My journey back to self, turned out to be the impetus for my life's work: teaching people to explore and trust their inner wisdom so they can live more authentically and fully.

The inspiration behind this book stems from my story, but also more than 40 years of intense self-reflection and exploration. Honestly, when I reflect, I realize I've been on a path of inner wisdom my entire life.

I came to mindfulness with a writer, English professor, and educator's mind. As a community college instructor for more than 25 years, the heart of my work is encouraging students to discover their passion. Before then, as a journalist, editor, community organizer and freelance writer, I was dedicated to speaking the truth and getting to the heart of things.

Over the course of more than 40 years, I developed a growth-mindset process that has helped me regain trust in myself and live more authentically. I wrote this book to not only share my 5-step method for growth but also to teach people how to have more clarity, reclaim focus, and cultivate more productivity and passion for life.

This book is an interactive roadmap to help people discover the hidden wisdom within themselves. It is a personal guide to fuel inner wisdom and self-acceptance. More importantly, these practices are accessible and potentially powerful for anyone; you don't have to be traditionally educated or well-versed in personal growth to begin this journey.

In short, this book and the inclusive 5-step method within it will give readers the tools to begin their own transformative journeys to self-discovery and living fully.

I know from personal experience that it's possible for *anyone* to tap into this practice. I've done it, and I continue to do it daily through various mindfulness techniques, adaptive chair yoga, and deep, exploratory journal writing.

It's taken more than 40 years to develop my 5-step exploration method, and I still rely heavily on these practices; they have shaped and helped me reclaim inner wisdom and regain balance in my life.

The good news is that you don't have to be a yogi to integrate mindfulness practices into your life. The simple, beautiful, and accessible practices in this book are designed to help you reduce stress, regain presence, and reconnect with your own inner wisdom and authenticity no matter who you are or where your interests lie.

In other words, mindful awareness can transform your life. I know; I've experienced it. And I'm honored to guide you on your own journey to authenticity.

The heart of my message is that we each have the capacity to learn and grow and experience life more fully.

Mindful Practice: A Beginner's Guide to Vibrant Living is for anyone going through a transition or life crisis, or who is interested in reinvigorating their life or unearthing more passion. This book is for anyone who has felt overwhelmed, on the verge of burnout, or burdened by life, personal challenges, or adversity.

It's also for people who have never been exposed to mindful practice but are interested in an introduction to mindful tools to improve their life. It will inspire, encourage, educate, and empower you to tap into and use your own inner wisdom and live a more authentic version of yourself.

We each already possess everything we need right now to find and live our own personal truth. With these tools, you can awaken and experience that truth. Because when we relax, listen, feel, embrace, and accept what comes, any one of us can be the hero of our own life. Growth is within reach when we trust ourselves. You already know the way.

Getting Started

The truth of who we are lies within us. We don't have to seek help outside ourselves to find the truth of who we are. We already have everything we need right now—all we need to do is learn to tap into our inner wisdom—our own personal inner guide knows what to do.

I came to this realization after more than 40 years of deep exploration and self-reflection. My path was truly revealed after I survived a devastating car accident at 19 years old and was diagnosed with a spinal cord injury. Before the accident, I was a dancer and choreographer with dreams of performing on Broadway. Afterward, I felt as though my world had collapsed. I had little hope for my future. When I awoke in the hospital, a week later, doctors said I wouldn't walk again. I was paralyzed, numb with no feeling or sensation in various parts of my body below my hips, knees, and feet. I was stunned. I couldn't believe this reality. I became determined to prove them wrong. I built a wall around my emotions and disconnected from my body. At the time, self-protection kept me alive. I became obsessed with pushing through difficulties and hiding weaknesses. When doctors and health professionals told me I would never be able to walk, I resisted. My defiance made me resilient, yet I had only touched the surface of my inner truth.

What I didn't know or wasn't able to see back then was that the trauma of my car accident was a gateway to deeper growth. I had everything I needed, but I didn't know how to reveal it.

And so, after the accident, I fed my mind and body with external truths. I thought if I pushed myself and my body as hard as possible,

I could prove my worth. Even though I was repeatedly told I wouldn't walk again, I was determined to do it.

After a year and a half of intense physical therapy, I didn't regain sensation or feeling below my hips, knees, and feet, but I progressed from a wheelchair to using forearm crutches and then a cane for support. By some miracle, I relearned to walk with foot orthotics, but this was a long and painful process and only the beginning of my journey back to self. Nevertheless, it's what gave me the confidence to rebuild my life. I'm still grateful for the many doctors and health professionals who helped me, but no one back then could see that I was truly struggling within.

On the outside, I felt strong, but my inner world was in turmoil. I always had a strong intuition as a child, but somehow the car accident had stripped away my internal confidence. Relearning to walk was the first step to healing, but in other ways, I had a long way to go. The trauma of the accident had shut down the deep connection I've always had with my mind and my body. This disconnection from my inner truth felt like a betrayal. My journey to self has been a long one, but along the way I discovered the power of inner wisdom. And I'm grateful to share my 5-step exploratory method that stemmed from that wisdom with you.

5-Step Exploration Method

As mentioned earlier in the book, the heart of my message is that we each have the capacity to learn and grow and experience life more fully. My daily mindfulness journey stems from my work as an adaptive, accessible chair yoga teacher, but the interactive practices in this book can transfer to anyone; you don't have to be educated in personal growth to begin this work.

Mindful Practice offers 25 inspirational mantras and quotes, inclusive interactive exercises, and journal writing to jumpstart self-awareness and power your life. Each section includes 5 chapters and highlights my 5-step exploration method. The chapters begin with an inspirational mantra or affirmation and quote, inclusive, mindful body movement or yoga pose, and an exploratory journal prompt for deep reflection.

The inspirational mantras and quotes are followed by paragraphs to introduce the concept or idea. An inclusive, mindful awareness practice provides direction, which leads to an exploratory writing prompt. Overall, this hands-on book is for the layperson seeking balance and personal growth.

As mentioned earlier, it's taken more than 40 years to develop my 5-step exploration method, but, for me, these steps have been a gateway that helped me reclaim inner wisdom and regain balance in my life.

The following steps are the method I used to reclaim my life. You may find it useful to walk through the pages in this book in order, but feel free to explore or skip around and adapt for yourself. There is no one way to begin. This is *your* journey: I encourage you to remain open to what's revealed.

Step 1: Relax.

In this step, try to release tension and constraints in the mind, body, and spirit. Let go of all distractions. Focus on now.

Step 2: Listen.

In this step, tap into your inner knowing, understanding and empathy for yourself and your mind, body, and spirit.

Step 3: Feel.

In this step, try to identify what physical and emotional sensations come up in your practice and embody these sensations in your mind, body, and spirit.

Step 4: Embrace.

In this step, integrate your inner knowing or inner state of being and allow it to open your mind, body, and spirit.

Step 5: Accept.

In this step, try to receive and welcome the gift of the present moment with ease and self-compassion. Trust that what's revealed feeds your whole being or your mind, body, and spirit.

Mindful Practice

The inclusive, mindful practices in this book provide an adaptable, accessible approach to mindfulness and movement. Since I'm an adaptive chair yoga teacher, the movement practices focus on chair yoga; however, many of the practices can be done on the floor on a yoga mat if needed or preferred.

As when beginning any new program, it's important to listen to your body and adapt or omit any movements that don't feel good. If you feel tension, strain, pull, pain, or throbbing in a practice, come out of the practice, back to neutral center or center, and breathe. I like to begin my practice in prayer pose or hands together resting at heart center, which I often refer to as heart center in the book. But again, you have many neutral and center options to choose from, which we'll explore in detail later.

As far as equipment, you may want to purchase one or two yoga blocks to support your practice. But a DIY method could be to use large soup cans in place of yoga blocks or practice near a wall. Again, you may or may not use a yoga mat in mindful practice—and since I practice adaptive chair yoga, there are days when I don't use a mat. Sometimes I pick any chair in my house and practice. I don't put constraints on mindful practice. And you don't have to purchase anything or join a gym to start this journey. The practices in this book can be completed anytime, anywhere; it's an interactive jumping-off point.

Additionally, while many say mindful practice must be done barefoot, this is not required in my view. I don't take my shoes off for mindful practice because I have physical challenges and need my shoes to walk. But again, play around with what works for you.

The point is: you don't need to purchase fancy clothes or equipment if it doesn't fit your budget. Try and see what feels right for you. This is your journey; make it accessible and fun.

Remember, you are the engineer—the most important teacher in the room. Trust your instincts and listen to your body, always. Customize what's best for you.

Your mindful practice is your own.

How to Use Mantras

Mindful practitioners use mantras and affirmations to calm and center the mind and body. In general, mantras are often referred to as sounds that carry vibration to help you locate harmony with the world or universe. Affirmations are positive phrases that help you reset old mindsets. I'm using the terms (mantras and affirmations) together in this book merely as an introduction to both. There is no one method for choosing a word, phrase, idea, or chant that works for you. To benefit from such a practice, you will want to repeat the phrase many times. Some say 108 is the magic number. My advice: experiment—find out what works for you.

You may also find that repeating a mantra or affirmation pairs nicely with meditation or mindful practice. Either way, the purpose of this book is to provide integrative tools for you to use in your life. Try them out and pick and choose what feeds your journey.

Just like using our breath to center and calm the mind, using mantras and affirmations anchor us in the present moment. Using both tools can change perspective and become the grounding force to mindful practice and meditation. A mantra or affirmation can reach your consciousness and bring you back to your inner wisdom. Again, pick and choose which tools help you feel whole. Or create some of your own. The point is to dive in and experiment.

So, let's get started on your journey. Friendly reminder: you may walk through each section in order or skip around if you like. Either way, you hold the key to your progress. Follow your inner compass. You know the way.

Relax

Section One: *Relax*

Chapter 1
Mantra: I am strong.

"Women are like teabags. We don't know our true strength until we are in hot water."

Eleanor Roosevelt

"You look normal sitting down. It's only when you start to walk that we notice your limp," my therapist said.

"Why would she say that?" I asked myself. Having a limp didn't make me abnormal. Her statement made me question myself. It hurt my self-esteem. I wasn't in therapy to talk about my limp or my spinal cord injury, which occurred because of a car accident when I was 19. I started therapy to deal with the death of my stepdad Mark. He had helped me face life after surviving a devastating car accident. But instead of addressing my therapist's off-putting remark, I ignored it and stuffed my feelings.

When I was a child, I was taught that if someone hurts you, it's best to rise above it. I was also taught that when faced with adversity (or if you want something badly enough) it's up to you to work hard and make it happen. On the surface, these may seem sensible, but ultimately, they are limiting beliefs that keep us stuck.

It took me a long time to unravel both mindsets, but eventually I discovered that we don't have to strive or struggle through difficulty to improve our lives. Adversity can make us stronger, but it's only one small part of the growth-work puzzle.

In fact, embracing the mess (and vulnerability) is where the beauty lies. It's a pathway to joy.

But this lesson didn't unfold easily.

Before the car accident, I felt invincible. I was physically strong and never gave up on my goals. As a dancer, athlete, lifeguard, cheerleader, and choreographer, I knew who I was and what I wanted to do with my life after high school: go to New York to become a Broadway dancer and choreographer.

After the accident, I lost my sense of self. I struggled with limited mobility and lack of sensation; it felt like torture. When you're an athlete or a dancer, your body is your instrument; if that instrument no longer plays as it once did, your connection to it is broken, and it's very easy to feel ungrounded. My dreams were shattered; my connection with my body forever changed. I had no idea how to heal. It took a long time to reclaim the power within myself, find compassion, and create a new life with new dreams.

Healing came in pieces over 40 years, as I developed an exploration process to reconnect with my body and find self-compassion.

Below is a mindful practice that grounds and expands my sense of self. I use *Mountain Pose* to destress and awaken inner wisdom.

Mindful Practice:

Mountain Pose

*Sit in a chair with your feet on the floor (or elevated on yoga blocks or pillows or blankets if your feet don't reach the floor).

*Legs should be hip distance apart in a relaxed state.

*Rock back and forth on your sitting bones to find a comfortable seated position.

*Soften and relax your shoulders down, away from your ears to help your neck and upper back muscles relax.

*Center your head in line with your spine and relax your arms alongside your body on both sides of your chair.

*Or you could bring your hands together in front of your heart (or at heart center) in Namaste or prayer position if that feels good.

*Gently ground down through your feet, anchoring all four corners of each foot into the floor or blocks.

*This anchoring can help you engage your legs so you really can feel the stability of this pose and the strength in your body.

*Breathe in and out of your nose for further grounding and relax into this sensation.

*Try a few rounds of breath in and out of your nose. You can increase the rounds of breath as your practice expands. If you feel dizzy at any point, stop and rest.

*Close your eyes (and soften your gaze) and bring awareness to your body. Let your mind rest. Relax with each breath.

*This is a power pose or seated *Tadasana* or *Mountain Pose*.

*When you come out of the pose, prepare to answer the following prompt.

Exploratory Writing Prompt: The key to personal growth is exploration. How have you used exploration in your life? Think of a time when you explored. Describe the situation and how you felt. Where can you be more adventurous in your life?

Chapter 2
Mantra: Relax, the world is working in my favor.

"We will be more successful in all our endeavors if we can let go of the habit of running all the time, and take little pauses to relax and recenter ourselves. And we'll also have a lot more joy in living."
Thich Nhat Hanh

Our lives travel in many directions, but mindfulness teaches that no matter what happens or what circumstances we face—the world is working in our favor. I've come to know this deeply in my adaptive chair yoga practice, but also as an online educator.

Since I teach college English online and work from home, one of the most important lessons I've learned is to schedule rest. It's a challenge when students can reach us anytime via email. But we do ourselves a disservice when we don't make time to replenish mind, body, and soul.

No matter what comes up in my life, I embrace the truth that everything is working in my favor. When things don't go my way, I resist the temptation to mourn what doesn't work because I realize all things that are meant for me will come in due time. I was raised to have a strong spiritual understanding that life has my back. There are storms, of course, but this belief fills me with hope, and that keeps me from chasing after people or things.

The following practice can center your entire being and help you connect with your inner guide. Taking a deep, mindful sigh every day can clear out the cobwebs and make space for significant personal growth.

Mindful Practice:

Sigh-out Breath

**Sigh-out Breath* can bring a sense of relaxation to both mind and body.

*Sit tall in a chair. Gaze straight ahead, relax your shoulders and settle in.

*Find a hand position that feels good to you, palms up on your thighs, or perhaps resting under your belly or where your belly and thighs meet.

*Wiggle your fingers to release tension in your fingertips, feeling stress fall away with each wiggle.

*Inhale through your nose, filling your lungs to full capacity.

*Exhale sigh-out your breath with your mouth open, making a *Ha* sound in the back of your throat.

*Do a couple more rounds of breath like this.

*Inhale through your nose, exhale out with a big sigh through your mouth.

*Feel your body relax more with each breath.

*When you inhale, say *"let"* to yourself.

*When you exhale, say *"go"* to yourself.

*Deepen this relaxation by closing your eyes. If closing your eyes doesn't feel good, try a relaxed gaze, or focus eyes on something across the room.

*Enjoy the mind, body connection.

*When ready, answer the following prompt.

Exploratory Writing Prompt: Do you share your hopes and dreams with others? Why or why not? Where have you participated in separation instead of connection? Have you made yourself small to fit in? How can you root in compassion for yourself and others?

Chapter 3
Mantra: Follow higher self.

"I have learned that as long as I hold fast to my beliefs and values—and follow my own moral compass—then the only expectations I need to live up to are my own."
Michelle Obama

The biggest gift of my car accident was learning to face my fear of being seen. After the accident, I wanted to hide. Remaining invisible fed my fear of being viewed as disabled. Even though I walk with a limp—I thought that if I relearned to walk, I wouldn't be disabled; this flawed thinking filtered my experiences, which led to limiting beliefs. For example, I used to say, "Who am I if I'm not a dancer? I don't know what to do with my life."

With age and maturity, I realized every challenge—no matter how big or small—was an opportunity to embrace my whole self. We become resilient when we embrace all facets of life: wins, losses, and everything in between. More importantly, we don't have to push, strive, or work ourselves to death to find happiness. We also don't have to hide our pain or our feelings or rise above our circumstances to survive trauma. And even though our journeys may feel separate from those of others, our diverse stories are beautiful—our human flaws connect us. There's a treasure trove of gifts beneath our challenges; reframing this for myself opened my world.

Chair Centering or *Grounding* is one tool that opens my heart to my higher self. For me, it feels like I'm following my moral compass; in this space I need only live up to my own expectations.

Mindful Practice:

Chair Centering or *Grounding*

*Sit in a chair, in a comfortable position, with your spine long.

*Feel your sitting bones connect with the chair. Relax and feel the weight of the chair seat supporting you.

*Focus on this feeling of support as you ground your body to the chair.

*Rock your body side to side to settle in further.

*Once settled, rest your hands palms up on your knees, thighs, or back against the belly.

*Find a comfortable hand position that feels right for you.

*Take a slow, deep belly breath in and out through your nose.

*Release tension in your body as you find this centering breath.

*Let go of all tension, holding, or constricting in your body.

*As you relax, continue to elongate spine and sit tall in your chair.

*As you inhale, say to yourself, *"relax."*

*As you exhale, say to yourself, *"follow higher self."*

*If it feels good, close your eyes to deepen relaxation. If closing your eyes, doesn't feel good, soften your gaze on something across the room.

*If your mind starts to wander, focus on your breath, and say the words above to yourself.

*Center like this for 5-10 minutes daily. You can do this in the early morning or before bedtime, or anytime you can carve out a bit of time for it. You can even do this in the bathroom at work, or at an airport, or anytime you need to reset.

*Set a timer (if that feels helpful) so you can feel sensation without interruption.

*You can build up to more time as your practice develops.

*Center yourself.

*Ground.

*Relax.

*When ready, answer the following prompt.

Exploratory Writing Prompt: Who have I always admired? Try to pick someone you know and have a relationship with. If no one comes to mind, you may pick someone famous. Focus on the qualities this person holds that you admire, as opposed to their achievements or status. What makes that person special? Now, ask yourself and write down your answer to the following question: *how can I reflect more of those qualities in my life and relationships?*

Chapter 4
Mantra: I am enough.

"Be thankful for what you have; you'll end up having more. If you concentrate on what you don't have, you will never, ever have enough."

Oprah Winfrey

When I was in graduate school, I was a cultural studies major with an emphasis on women in film. In simple terms, I was a film nerd with a penchant for independent cinema (I still am). In addition to being a Graduate Teaching Assistant in the English department, graduate school brought much self-discovery. I found a lifelong passion for teaching; I loved sharing information and connecting with others.

Some of my favorite classes to attend were film seminars, and one favorite centered on Director Alfred Hitchcock; it was called, *Framing Hitchcock*. Another favorite seminar focused on Director Stanley Kubrick, and this led to an opportunity to participate in a film panel at a cultural studies conference in Iowa. Our topic was male subjectivity, and my focus was Kubrick's *A Clockwork Orange*. Soaking up academia and participating in conferences fed my desire for knowledge and guided me to discover my passion for writing film reviews.

When I was working on my bachelor's degree, I wrote film reviews for my college newspaper, where I was editor. When I was accepted into grad school at another college across the state, I had to start over and find a new place to publish reviews. Securing this gig wasn't easy.

First, I was the only female freelance reviewer on staff. In fact, the editor said during our first meeting, "We've never had a female reviewer," as if it were a disease. I had to prove myself on several occasions. Mainly, I had to play by the "old boy's network" rules to get published.

Internally, I hated the politics of this game, but I stuck with it because I thought writing reviews was my calling. Therefore, I freelanced for this newspaper for several years while in graduate school. Eventually, I moved on when it was clear I could no longer choose the type of films I wanted to review.

But a wonderful thing happened. Letting go of my freelance writing job led to new opportunities. After earning my master's degree, I took a low-paying but extremely fulfilling job as a breast cancer awareness coordinator, where I worked on a federal grant to help uninsured women get free mammograms. I traveled to 18 Kansas counties, gave presentations, wrote tons of articles and PR material, and met many wonderful people. It replenished my heart and soul. I loved this job.

My point: making choices may not be easy, but it opens the door to new things. I no longer fear when doors close. I realize a new window will open, and that will lead to new adventures.

The following breathwork practice works wonderfully as a regular mediative tool or for anytime you want to quiet your mind and find more balance in your life. This type of breathwork can relax the body and reduce stress and anxiety. Some experts say it can also lower heart rate, and over time, improve overall health and well-being.

Mindful Practice:

Alternate Nostril Breath

*To begin, sit comfortably in your chair.

*With the left hand resting comfortably on your left knee, lift your right hand toward your nose.

*Exhale completely, then use the right thumb to close your right nostril as you inhale through your left nostril.

*Inhale through the left nostril and then close the left nostril with your right index or middle finger.

*Open the right nostril and exhale through this side.

*Inhale through the right nostril and then close this nostril.

*Open the left nostril and exhale through the left side.

*This is one cycle.

*Continue alternate nostril breath for 2-5 minutes. If you feel dizzy, stop and rest.

*Start with 2 cycles and then try 2 minutes if you're new to this practice; it takes time to build up to 5 minutes.

*Start slow.

*Complete the practice by finishing with an exhale on the left side.

*This practice rejuvenates the mind and body and helps tap into inner peace. It can be done anytime, anywhere you need an energy uplift.

*When ready, answer the following prompt.

Exploratory Writing Prompt: Where do you find peace in your body? Describe the sensation with gratitude, focus on and appreciate what you take for granted. Now, consider where you feel energized in your life. How can you bring that energy into every day or the present moment?

Chapter 5
Mantra: Relax and trust.

"The most common way people give up their power is by thinking they don't have any."
Alice Walker

I was raised in a white, middle-class two-parent household in a quiet, middle-sized Kansas town. When I was 17, my parents divorced, and my simple, familiar world was altered. I went from having everything a typical privileged white girl had grown accustomed to shuffling between two separate households and living on a budget.

But there were also many wonderful, unexpected gifts that stemmed from this change. When my parents each remarried, I gained two new families; both brightened my world—love and laughter connected us. I also found joy in connecting with my boyfriend (now husband's) family. I loved hearing and sharing family stories in all three households; these new and meaningful relationships nurtured me. In fact, my husband's sisters teased him daily by saying, "We love Mary more than you."

Being part of a fun-loving clan that loves us unconditionally builds a strong foundation. There's nothing like feeling whole, nourished, and embraced for who we are.

In less than two years, however (when the car accident occurred) I discovered cracks in my foundation. When diagnosed with a spinal cord injury (SCI), I lost my Dad's health insurance because it was considered a preexisting condition. Therefore, I was on my own without health coverage.

Few doctors were willing to treat someone with a preexisting condition in the 1980s, and many turned me away. If I had a health issue, I went to the emergency room, where I couldn't pay for the services. As a result, I often went without care and felt demoralized for needing help. It was a vicious cycle. Yet, somewhere, deep down, I knew all this was preparation for something more.

I tried to gain strength when well-meaning friends and family said, "what doesn't kill you makes you stronger," but bitterness crept in. At times, I imagined I was a female Charlie Brown, who felt overwhelmed with limited options. In the words of my Grandma and Mom, I was "on the pity pot." I longed for ease, but it was difficult to find because I was rejecting the reality of my now limited mobility.

As a feminist and a former dancer, I thought I had control over my body, but the accident undermined my autonomy. I now felt betrayed by my body. I beat myself up constantly. Mainly, I didn't know how to ask for help.

I was able to find some relief when I started practicing *Lion's Breath*. This practice not only empowers me, but it also energizes my whole being. It's a wonderful, mindful reset to connect with the present moment. Give it a try and see if it releases the lion within you!

Mindful Practice:

Lion's Breath Variation

*To begin, sit comfortably in a chair with your legs shoulder width.

*Find the center in your seat, rock back and forth, and place your palms firmly against your knees or thighs.

*You can spread your fingers out like lion claws if you like.

*Set your gaze forward at either the tip of your nose or between your eyebrows.

*Inhale deeply through the nose, then open mouth wide, stick tongue out and curl it down as you deeply exhale, making an extended *Ha* sound. (You can even roar if you want to!)

*Feel the muscles in the face contract and your throat muscles tighten as you inhale and exhale.

*Open your eyes extremely wide as you exhale.

*The point of this practice is to lighten up, relax, and awaken your inner lion.

*Now, when ready, prepare to answer the following prompt.

Exploratory Writing Prompt: Write about a time when you felt alive and awake in your life. Share as many descriptive details as you can recall sparking your imagination. Devote 5-10 minutes of uninterrupted writing. Set a timer, so there's no need to lift the pen from the page. When the timer sounds, look at what you've written. Circle what feels important. Now, ask yourself: *where can you bring more awareness in your life? If it awakens the lion in you, how does this feel? Why is this important?*

Listen

Section Two: *Listen*

Chapter 6
Mantra: I'll be Ok - no matter what.

"Cultivate the habit of being grateful for every good thing that comes to you, and to give thanks continuously. And because all things have contributed to your advancement, you should include all things in our gratitude."

Ralph Waldo Emerson

One way to open and connect the mind, body, and heart is to cultivate a practice of gratitude. I started a gratitude journal years ago, and it truly helps me connect with "simple abundance," a term attributed to best-selling author, philanthropist, and public speaker Sarah Ban Breathnach. Theologians also speak of the power of gratitude, but I think it's deeper than that.

When we're grateful for the simple things, we don't want what we don't have. Our life feels full and seemingly mundane moments take on profound meaning.

Experts say self-awareness is the gateway to growth. I agree. When we know ourselves fully, we can recognize our blind spots but also become our own best champion. Being thankful for the smallest moment can open your heart and mind to a whole new world of gratitude. And this increased awareness can lead us to better decisions and help us to eliminate bad habits.

The following practice can clear your mind of clutter in preparation for self-reflection. A useful companion practice I find is to keep track of my inner voice. You might try this as well. Listen to the words you say to yourself each day. Is your inner critic telling you that you're not good enough?

Some experts say that learning to speak positively to ourselves and others on a regular basis has a direct correlation between higher living and self-awareness. Keep a log of what you say to yourself in times of stress or overwhelm. Then, work on changing those ingrained patterns. Can you replace the criticism with compassion? Can you speak to yourself with the same care and understanding that you would a dear friend who was struggling? Be kind to yourself. Feed your internal world.

Mindful Practice:

Cultivate Gratitude Body Stretch

* Sit tall in your chair, rest your hands softly on top of your thighs, and ground down through your feet.

* Close your eyes if that helps you turn inward.

* Take in a few deep, mind-clearing/cleansing breaths in and out of your nose.

* When you're ready, move your hands to rest alongside you on both sides of your chair, and on an inhale, reach your arms above and then slightly behind your head.

* Be sure to listen to your body and let up on movement if you feel strain.

* You may arch back slightly and move your head up if this feels good. But be mindful of what messages your body is sending; if you feel strain, pain, or any pulling, let up on movement.

*On exhale, release arms back to resting position alongside your chair.

*_Variation_: I like to place a pillow behind my back for support. Play around with your setup to find what feels good to you.

*While in this stretch, take a few cleansing breaths—listening to how your body responds.

*While breathing—ask yourself: _what am I grateful for or how can I bring more gratitude into my life?_ Phrase the question so it makes sense to you or make up your own phrase.

*On an exhale, release your arms and come back to neutral, returning your hands to rest on top of your thighs.

*Repeat the gratitude stretch with a few rounds of nostril breath.

*After a few rounds, bring your hands to rest at your heart center for a moment and prepare to answer the following prompt.

Exploratory Writing Prompt: What are you grateful for in your life, and how can you bring more gratitude into your life? Write down three things you're grateful for—they can be as small or large as you like. Don't censor yourself. Search your mind for what fills you up with gratitude. Feel free to use this practice and prompt daily. It's a wonderful reset.

Chapter 7
Mantra: I am thriving. I am playful.

"My mission in life is not merely to survive, but to thrive; and to do so with some passion, some compassion, some humor, and some style."

Maya Angelou

Maya Angelou has saved my life many times, especially her poem, *Still I Rise,* which begins:

"You may write me down in your history

With your bitter, twisted lies

You may trod me in the very dirt

But still, like dust, I rise."

Her work fills me with resilience. There is nothing that can crush our spirit if we believe in ourselves. When we create space to find our voice, we can truly thrive. One way I do this is to stay playful and look for places in my day to feel joy. Playing piano, listening to music, and creating groovy duct-taped crafts feels my heart with joy. And some health professionals say laughing therapy or even just a deep belly laugh can invigorate and brighten your mood; I practice this every day because it not only lifts my spirits—but it also helps me lighten up when life gets messy.

Another way to feel joyful is to infuse fun into your regular routine; and for me, that means finding creative ways to move my body. Feel free to create your own variation of the following practice, incorporating any movements that make you feel joyful. When we become open, it can manifest within us as joy, fulfillment, and a sense of higher purpose.

Mindful Practice:

Playful Movement

*You can do this practice seated or standing, pick what feels best.

*Ground down feet for stability. Feel four corners of your feet as you ground.

*Circle your arms one at a time and move with breath, breathing in and out through your nose if possible.

* Begin by grounding feet on the floor. Inhale as you sweep up your right arm forward and up. Exhale, twist, or turn your torso to the right and gaze back slightly as your arm swims behind you.

*If you're seated, it will likely look as though you're doing a seated backstroke.

*Keep going, moving one arm and then the other.

*Move with breath, breathe in and out through your nose.

*Keep the circle flows slow and easy.

*ptop*Variation*: Lift or circle your arms one at a time but omit the twist.

*Feel free to play here! Try moving your arms up, down, and around in random movements, much like a ballet movement.

*Remember: this is meant to be fun and energizing, but this isn't a race.

*This is your practice. Customize it however you like.

*Explore how this feels in your body.

*Be mindful. Go steady and slow.

*Keep breathing. Feel awareness of your body.

*On the last exhale, return to your center and bring your hands into prayer position.

*This is your heart center.

*Take a few cleansing breaths in and out through your nose.

*When ready, answer the following prompt.

Exploratory Writing Prompt: When was the last time you had fun? When was the last time you took an unplanned or spontaneous road trip? Describe the scenario. Then, think about ways that you might bring more play into your life. Write down some ideas you'd like to implement.

Chapter 8
Mantra: Trust yourself.

"You, yourself, as much as anyone in the entire universe, deserve your love and affection."

Buddha

Self-care is a crucial part of my life. Self-care can be defined as anything that nourishes, replenishes, soothes, or calms our whole being. For me, self-care is how I maintain balance.

We all have our favorite ways to take care of ourselves. I use meditation, yoga, journaling, music, and crafting. Whether your self-care choices are similar or different, the point is that self-care doesn't need to be extravagant; it can be engaging in simple pleasures—things that bring us happiness and joy. Though they're simple, they're important because they help make life meaningful. Give yourself permission to do what makes you happy. When we live our passion effortlessly, we find new ways to trust ourselves without pushing or striving.

The following practice is a wonderful way to embrace radical self-love. It is a gentle reminder to set aside time for yourself. If you feel guilt around engaging in self-care, remember that it's difficult to give to others when your reserve is empty. Replenishing ourselves helps us trust our choices, which is the first step to wholeness.

Mindful Practice:

Seated Push-Up

*Bring your chair to face a wall.

*Leave enough room between the chair and wall for your hands to comfortably touch it when your elbows are bend and straight.

*_Variation_: If standing is available and comfortable for you, you can stand facing the wall instead.

*Place hands on the wall shoulder-width, arms straight.

*On an inhale, bend your elbows for a push-up.

*On exhale, extend your arms to press back up.

*Do 5-10 rounds or whatever feels good for your practice.

*No need to rush; move slowly and mindfully and continue to pair your movement with your breath.

*_Variation_: Move arms past shoulder width and try a push in this position with breath.

*When you're finished, answer the following prompt.

Exploratory Writing Prompt: What do you want out of life? In what ways can you trust that life will work in your favor? How can you make this a reality without pushing or striving? Is it possible to let things reveal themselves on their own? If so, how would this feel?

Chapter 9
Mantra: I am grateful to be alive.

"We can only be said to be alive in those moments when our hearts are conscious of our treasures."

Thornton Wilder

Some people refer to inner wisdom as inner connection. No matter what you call it, learning to cultivate inner wisdom can bring more ease and gratitude into your life.

In his book, *The Teacher Appears: 108 Prompts to Power Your Yoga Practice,* Brian Leaf describes inner wisdom as something that can be "a calm, serene feeling or a passionate, electric feeling" and "a deep sense of rightness." Living from this "rightness" can be liberating says Leaf because "you're not chained to pretense or restricted by keeping up some facade."

Leaf also suggests that we can reprogram the brain to live from a sense of what feels right for us. He goes on to say that since we all have cellphones nowadays, we can use our phones to reprogram our brain to listen to our inner wisdom. That is, "every time we hear a beep or buzz, stop what you're doing and take a deep, relaxing breath." Adding this to your daily routine can have a positive effect on your ability to decrease stress and increase gratitude.

Below is another helpful, deeply heart-centered inner wisdom exercise you can do anywhere. *Seated Inner Connect* has certainly made a difference in my life.

Mindful Practice:

Seated Inner Connect

*Sit in a chair with elongated spine, your back away from the chair (if this feels good to you), and feet planted firmly on the floor.

*If you feel strain in this neutral seated position, sit back in the chair for more support.

*Find what's comfortable and prepare to listen.

*Flex and extend your hands and your fingers a few times, then rest your hands on your thighs, and breathe in and out through your nose.

*Bring both hands to your heart and stack them on top of each other.

*Then relax your facial muscles, throat, and neck, and continue to breathe.

*Listen deep into your heart. . .can you feel a sense of ease radiate from your heart center?

*Picture a warm, soothing light emanating from the inside of your heart—can you feel an accompanying sense of calm as you breathe in and out through your nose?

*Visualize this light expanding, filling your heart as you continue to breathe.

*Let the expansiveness feeling calm your inner spirit.

*Now, close your eyes (if that feels good) or soften your gaze, and linger in this luxurious space for a few minutes.

*Use this practice anytime or anywhere.

*For me, it decreases stress, anxiety, and feelings of overwhelm.

*This is inner wisdom—*this is how to tap into your inner guide.*

*Make a gentle transition back to neutral seated position and open your eyes slowly.

*When ready, answer the following prompt.

Exploratory Writing Prompt: We all know we are alive, but in what ways have you felt truly alive in the last month? Describe a situation where you felt energized by life. If you're unable to locate one, envision a scenario that would allow you to feel energized. What does it look like? Is someone else with you, or are you alone? Write for 5 minutes about how this feels in your body. Try to include some of the five senses (sight, smell, taste, touch, and sound) as you listen to the sensations and cues from your body. How can you cultivate this energized feeling at least once every day?

Chapter 10
Mantra: Listen with curiosity.

"Most people do not listen with the intent to understand; they listen with the intent to reply."

Stephen R. Covey

According to my Mom, I was an extremely shy child and preferred watching and listening instead of talking. This concerned my parents, but there was a logical reason for my choice. It was partly because my older Brother fetched me anything I wanted. There was no need to ask. All I had to do was point, and he retrieved it. If I was in room of strangers, and he was absent, Mom said I would stare people down. I'd plant my "big, baby blues on someone," as Mom described it, and observed. No words, just deep, silent observation.

When my Brother started school, I was forced to talk to express my needs. And, I must admit, my desire for deep conversation has never since stopped. But as an adult, I remind myself to still take time to truly be present and listen.

Teaching ourselves to listen is a useful skill to pick up at any age. We need to quell the impulse to constantly share, which is difficult in a culture where oversharing is so common, especially on social media. If you have ever attended a lecture or a graduate school seminar, you know how hard it can be to sit down and shut up. But there is value in listening. It can even be empowering.

The same concept applies when it comes to listening to our inner selves. As children, we instinctively know what feels right for us. But when life happens, this gets harder; we realize we have so much to learn. Listening and being mindful are the first steps to living an empowered life. Keep in mind: we don't master these steps; it's an ongoing practice that evolves as we learn, change, and grow.

The mindful practices in this book are meant to jumpstart deep inner listening to provide an accessible gateway to personal growth. Once you create space to connect internally, the desire to seek outside acceptance may slowly diminish. Inner listening can cultivate curiosity and open our hearts and minds to the human condition, helping us to know ourselves more fully and find deep compassion for ourselves and others. The following practice is one of my favorites.

Mindful Practice:

Inner Listening

*Find a quiet spot to sit and clear your mind.

*Tap into your breath. Breathe in and out through your nose if possible.

*Notice how each inhale and exhale out of your nose brings you into deep inner listening.

*Once you find a centering rhythm, place your hands over your heart and continue breathing in and out of your nose.

*Close your eyes and relax all the parts of your body.

*You may wish to walk through the parts of your body one by one, inviting each to relax. You might say to yourself: *relax your toes. Relax your feet. Relax your ankles. Relax your knees. Relax your thighs*, and so on until you reach the top of your head.

*Allow the breath to cleanse and ease your mind and body.

*When you feel centered, ask yourself: *what do I need more of today?*

*Be open to the words that flow from your heart.

*Have a notepad ready to write down the message you receive.

*If nothing comes, stay centered and go deeper.

*It might help to say to yourself, *listen with curiosity.*

*Or create a mantra that feels right for you or pick one from this book to inspire your inner knowing to arise.

*After you have an answer, come out of silence slowly, open your eyes, then explore the following prompt.

Exploratory Writing Prompt: Think back to a time when you listened intently. How did that feel in your body? What sensations came up as you focused on a deep, heartfelt conversation? Does it feel calm, spacious, smooth, easy, soft, pleasurable, or light? Now, how can you bring more of this listening into all conversations? How would that feel?

Feel

Section Three: *Feel*

Chapter 11
Mantra: *I forgive those who have harmed me in my past and peacefully detach from them.*

"Happiness is not something ready-made. It comes from your own actions."

Dalai Lama

Three weeks after my car accident, I had a life-altering experience with one of my doctors. Overall, I had a team of wonderful doctors, but there was one who was unapproachable. Our relationship was strained from the start. He was curt, unavailable, and appeared irritated when I asked questions. My instincts about his character proved correct.

Just before I was scheduled to move to the physical rehabilitation hospital, he made a surprise visit one day and bluntly asked, "How does it feel to know you will never walk again?"

My jaw opened and my stomach dropped. His uncaring remark immediately made me defensive. No one had uttered anything like that to me. His words sucked the life out of my hope that I would walk again. Upon reflection, I now realize he was one of the catalysts for me relearning to walk. I turned my defiance into motivation and experienced a miracle when I was able to first walk with the aid of a wheelchair, then forearm crutches, and eventually a cane and two below-the-knee plastic braces.

I love how time and maturity reframed this experience for me. Once I learned to feel the pain of his words and peacefully detach from this experience, I reclaimed my power. Before then, my defiance determined my reaction. In time, I found that we all have the power to reframe disappointment and grow from it. I'm grateful for this encounter because it taught me to move past old wounds and heal.

I use the following pose, *Seated Cobra,* to reframe or shed old thinking. Since this pose activates the spine, I'm mindful of my back injury and what feels good in my body when I practice it. And even if you are injury free, the following pose can still help to decrease stiffness and increase flexibility by mobilizing the spine, and some say it can elevate mood.

I practice this pose every evening to shake off stress. As always, if you feel any pain, let up on movement. The goal is to feel good in your body. Forgive those who mean you harm; this is the path to enlightenment.

Mindful Practice:

Seated Cobra

*Place your hands on the chair seat on the sides, elbows back, and close to the body.

*As you hold the chair, inhale, raise up your head, neck, and chest toward the sky and bring your shoulders back and down. Arch your back slightly (if this feels good).

*You may find it feels good to scoot to the front edge of the chair and place hands on your knees or thighs but listen to your inner wisdom to find what setup works for you.

Variation: On an inhale, feel the opening of the chest. This time opt out of pressing on hands, but continue to raise up your head, neck and chest and bring your shoulders back and down.

*On an exhale, bring head, neck, and chest back to the starting position.

Variation: With hands alongside the chair, inhale and raise up head, neck, and chest then swing hands back (and head down) while extending arms past the back of the chair like a skier. Exhale back to the starting position.

*Again, listen to what feels good for your body.

*Do several rounds of this practice.

*When ready, answer the following prompt.

Exploratory Writing Prompt: Do you have close relationships that bring you joy? What do you want to activate in others? What actions can you take today to improve relationships that need mending? How would it feel to heal and improve relationships in your life?

Chapter 12
Mantra: My body is alive;
I feel mind, body, spirit.

"Yoga is the journey of the self, through the self, to the self."

The Bhagavad Gita

I have had the pleasure of working with many wonderful yoga teachers, mentors, and guides. Each brought something new into my practice. My yoga journey began when I met Jessa Baxter Peterson of Chapter Five Yoga in Manhattan, Kansas, and earned my 200-hour registered teaching certification through YogaWorks or RYT 200. Jessa was a wonderful teacher who taught her students how to listen to our bodies. She also kept a chair for me at her studio because she welcomed diversity and loved building community by making her classes welcoming for all her students. Jessa's kindness forever touched my heart. I also learned a great deal from working with yoga teacher Alexandria Crow, who taught me how to slow down movement and poses while supporting my spine injury.

My journey continued when I found an organization called Accessible Yoga via online search. It was such a thrill to find a community that believed yoga could be accessible for all, especially the disabled community. My passion led to attending the first Accessible Yoga Conference in Santa Barbara, California in 2015. Eventually, I took *Accessible Yoga Teacher Training* with founder Jivana Heyman. This led to meeting Matthew Sanford and taking Mind Body Solutions *Opening Yoga Instructor Training, Continuing Studies*, and *Mind Body Story Workshop.* My path continued to evolve when I took *Yoga for All Teaching Training* with Dianne Bondy and

Amber Karnes. All were wonderful experiences. All helped me find new ways to feel alive in mind, body, and spirit. The main thread that connects these trainings: learning to customize poses and realizing that we are the best teachers for our own bodies. Mostly, I learned that mindful practice is different for us all because we all live in different bodies with different challenges.

I carry this knowledge into my practice but also realize if we constantly fight against what our body needs, we won't feel the benefits of mindful practice, and even that is a lesson—because yoga and mindful practice are not about pushing our body to its limits or edge. At least for me, it's not about fitness; it's about taking a mindful approach to radical self-acceptance.

One favorite pose is the adaptive *Seated Side Angle*. This pose opens my hips and strengthens the back of my legs. I also like the deep, side-body stretch, which helps to increase flexibility in my spine. The result: when I add breath with side movement, I feel the power of the mind-body connection. When I focus on this feeling, I deeply connect to my body, and this sparks curiosity. Had I focused on what was too challenging or inaccessible for my body, I never would have found the pleasure of coming back into my body and giving it what it needed. Simple, focused movement with breath is enough. When we give our body what it needs and we embrace our true selves, we feed our whole being.

Mindful Practice:

Seated Side Angle

*From the seated chair position, open legs to chair width and ground down feet to the floor for support.

*With your spine tall, move your left arm and hold on to the left side of the chair.

*Inhale and lift your right arm up and overhead, even with your right ear.

*Keep shoulders down and relaxed.

*Feel the right side of the body stretch.

*Take a few rounds of breath, slowly in and out of your nose.

*No need to rush.

*Feel the sensation through your body while grounding feet down.

*You may close your eyes for deeper sensation or effect.

*Slowly bring your right arm down and return to the center or place your arm on your right thigh.

*Repeat the movement on the left side, making sure to breathe.

**Variation*: Interweave or clasp hands together in front of you and reach out in front with an inhale.

*You can bring your arms up as high as it feels good in your body; you can build up to bringing arms up above your head.

*Listen to your body.

*On exhale, return your arms to starting position.

**Variation*: Ground down feet and bring interwoven, clasped hands overhead with breath, but keep body facing forward.

*On inhale and clasped hands, slowly lean your body to the left.

*On exhale, slowly come back to arms centered overhead.

*Now, slowly lean your body to the right on inhale.

*On exhale, come back to arms centered overhead.

*Release your hands and return hands to your heart center.

*Take a few slow, cleansing breaths.

*When ready, answer the following prompt.

Exploratory Writing Prompt: Do you cultivate curiosity in your life? Share a story that demonstrates this. Delve into other ways to become more alive and aware in your mind, body, and spirit.

Chapter 13
Mantra: Just be you.

"Let yourself be drawn by the stronger pull of that which you truly love."

Rumi

After my car accident, I had no idea how to live with a spinal cord injury. I felt like my life was split in two: my body before and after the accident. Navigating my injury pushed me deeper into depression. The year and a half of intense physical therapy allowed me to walk with foot orthotics, but my relationship with my body was never the same.

Through much self-study and exploration, I discovered new passions and rediscovered some forgotten ones. First, I reconnected with my love of writing and developed an intense journaling practice. Then, I fell in love with journalism and teaching and pursued a bachelor's in journalism and master's degree in English. There were many fits and starts during this period. My truth was revealed when I discovered mindful practice and adaptive and accessible yoga. Developing a practice opened my world—I began to feel alive in my body and reconnected mind, body, and spirit.

You don't have to survive a car accident to begin again. Mindful practice is available to anyone. Anytime. Anywhere. No matter what the circumstance you're faced with, draw on the hope that all is not lost. We all can reconnect with ourselves and live more authentically. When we open to and are drawn to our passion, we find our true selves.

I love practicing *Seated Twist* because it reminds me to listen to my body. Being mindful of my injury keeps me present, but it also helps me connect to inner wisdom. Every part of my body is connected – I feel whole when I tap into this space.

Mindful Practice:

Seated Twist

*Move slightly forward in the chair.

**Variation*: Since I have a spine injury, I rest at the back of the chair for support.

*Explore what feels best for you.

*Always let your body decide when and how to move in and out of poses or mindful practice.

*Again, only you know what feels good in your body.

*Inhale and bring your left hand to the outside of your right thigh, the right hand behind you, or to your side with fingers pointing away.

*Elongate your spine slowly as you breathe.

*On an exhale, gently twist your torso, neck, and head to your right.

*With each inhale, elongate your spine, with exhale, see if you can twist a bit more without strain.

*Adjust the twist for your body and your practice.

*Don't go as far if you feel strain, dizziness, burning, throbbing, or pain.

*Listen to the messages your body shares with you.

*Customize your movement to fit your body and your practice.

*On exhale, bring head, neck, and torso back to starting position and take another deep breath in and out through your nose.

*Repeat the other side slowly.

*Observe the breath in seated twist.

*When you return to your center, take a couple of *Sigh-out Breaths* to refresh.

*Try practicing this pose two or three times or what feels good to your practice.

*When ready, answer the following prompt.

Exploratory Writing Prompt: What personal discoveries have brought you the most joy? What is your best attribute? What is your least favorite attribute? Name a highlight of the last month. What are you looking forward to next month? What would it feel like to just be you?

Chapter 14
Mantra: Feel, restore, keep hope alive.

"Hope is a thing that feathers, that perches in the soul, and sings the tune without the words, and never stops at all."

Emily Dickinson

My parents used to repeat a Bible verse to me when I was a child: when you're a child, you act as a child, but as an adult, we give up childish things. I understand why my parents shared this; they wanted to instill a sense of resilience that growing up is hard but necessary. Maturity is a choice. I appreciated the lesson—it taught me to accept what is front of me even when it's difficult. But I also believe that we need to hold space for the hope that although our lives may be hard, things will work out for the best. Being resilient doesn't mean giving up our hopes and dreams. For me, maturation means walking through our feelings and difficult times with dignity intact.

There is something dignified about practicing restorative poses like *Seated Child's Pose*. Besides reducing stress as you feel a passive stretch in the back, torso, hips, thighs, and ankles, this pose also reminds me that each phase of our life requires a new level of acceptance. Hope is important at every stage of life…I vow to stay in touch with my childhood innocence and accept what life offers. We need support from time to time, but when we tap into inner knowing, we can feel in our bones that all things work for the higher good.

Mindful Practice:

Seated Child's Pose

*Bring hands to the heart center and ground feet into the floor.

*Feel all four corners of your feet touch the floor. This provides balance and security for mindful practice.

*Now bring your arms alongside both sides of your chair.

*Let your arms hang—feel your stress release throughout your arms, your fingertips, and your entire body.

*On inhale, swing your arms up above your head.

*On exhale, swing your arms down towards your feet with head hanging down on your lap if that feels good.

*Hang there, breathe, relax, and feel your body. Take a couple rounds of nostril breath while you relax and feel.

*Rest your arms in a relaxed position along the floor and rest your stomach comfortably on top of your thighs (if this feels good).

*Rest forehead on legs (if this feels good) but don't strain.

*Find what feels good to you.

*Relax shoulders and neck in *Seated Child's Pose*.

*Do 5-10 rounds of breath as you rest comfortably and feel your body let go of all tension and constraints.

*To release the pose, slowly come back up and bring your arms to your heart center.

*Take a few rounds of cleansing breaths and feel the sensation of ease.

*When ready, answer the following prompt.

Exploratory Writing Prompt: Who do you go to when you need help, hope, and support? If you could tap into your inner wisdom right now, what does it say? Does it offer comfort, ease, or constraint? Do you listen to it? Why or why not?

Chapter 15
Mantra: My heart is open.

"I open my heart, knowing my love guides my every decision. All is well."

Louise Hay

This quote says it all. When we let love guide our decisions—love dwells within us. When our hearts are open, our life can unfold. The same can be said for creating mindful practice. I love to practice the following sequence. It opens my heart and connects all parts of my being. We all have inner wisdom, but the following practice can help you tap into your true self. For me, when my heart is open and I feel mind, body, and spirit—love abounds, and all is well.

Mindful Practice:

Seated Mini Sun Salute/Cat Cow Variation

*Repeat several rounds.

*Move slightly forward in the chair if this feels good to you.

**Variation*: Sitting at the back of the chair feels better for me since I have back issues. Customize movement for your body.

*Remember: adaptive chair yoga is for everyone.

*Listen to your body and adjust poses for your practice.

*Customize what feels best in your body.

*Give yourself permission to play. This makes chair yoga fun.

*When I say listen to your body, I want you to explore, play, and customize what feels good for your body in a pose.

*Always leave room to opt-out of anything.

*This is *your* mindful practice.

*Customize for yourself.

*Your practice is your own.

*Trust your instincts.

*Choose which back position feels good in your body for *Mini Sun Salute*.

*With legs hip distance or yoga block distance apart, come into a seated *Tadasana*.

*Shoulders are relaxed and down—not up around your neck.

*Center head and arms alongside the body or you can bring hands to your heart center in namaste or prayer position.

*Ground down your feet as you engage your legs.

*Feel the stability and strength of your body in this position. Breathe into this subtle sensation or breathe in and out through your nose.

*This is a power pose or seated *Tadasana* or *Mountain Pose*.

*Elongate spine, look forward, palms together in front of the chest at the heart center.

*Inhale, sweep or rise your arms overhead, stretch hands upward, as you relax your shoulders.

*On an exhale, hinge or lean forward from hips, lower chest toward thighs to chair forward fold. You may rest your arms near both sides of your feet if that feels good.

*Come down as far as comfortable for your body, round back, relax the head as your arms hang down or near the floor. No need to touch the floor unless this feels good to your body.

**Variation*: Put blocks in front to catch hands in forward fold.

*Then, on an inhale, bring hands halfway underneath knees with elongated spine and flat back, raise head, neck, and chest, pressing hands lightly below the knee if that feels good.

**Variation*: Try placing your hands on blocks.

*On an exhale, move body back down to the floor in a chair forward fold.

**Variation*: Use blocks to catch hands if that feels good.

*On an inhale, when you come back up, raise your right leg with knee bent, keep your spine long, put hands underneath thigh and hold your thigh it feels good.

*On an exhale, release your right leg down.

*Next, let's do seated *Cat Cow*.

*On an inhale, rest hands on top of thighs and knees as you raise up your head, neck, and chest, moving abdomen forward and tailbone down.

*On an exhale, come back into seated *Tadasana/Mountain Pose*, and take a few rounds of breath in and out through your nose.

*Inhale, raise up your arms overhead, then on exhale, lower back to seated chair with your hands at heart center.

*Now, repeat same movements and variations for the other leg.

*Repeat the sequence a few times, using breath with movement.

*Take a few rounds of breath with your hands at heart center.

*When ready, answer the following prompt.

Exploratory Writing Prompt: Write about a time when your heart was open, and you took a leap towards your dreams. How did you feel? Now, write about one thing you can do to work toward this reality. What mindset do you need to get there? How can you bring more of this into your life?

Embrace

Section Four: *Embrace*

Chapter 16
Mantra: I acknowledge my self-worth; my confidence is soaring. My life is just beginning.

"If your compassion doesn't include yourself, it is incomplete."

Jack Kornfield

Self-compassion is the key to a good life. Jack Kornfield's quote reminds me that our lives are not linear. No one is immune to making mistakes, but our experiences are important lessons; they open our world to acknowledge self-worth and new beginnings.

Maria Schriver's *I've Been Thinking* is a beautiful, wise book worth checking out. One favorite chapter talks about having the determination and imagination to follow your choices. Paying attention to our choices can lead to deep connection with our life purpose; it also affirms self-confidence.

At every turn, our lives can offer new beginnings, but we must start with self-compassion. The following practice reminds me that connecting mind and body creates compassion for my physical challenges. *Knee-to-Chest Awareness* improves circulation, but it also relaxes the mind and the body. For my practice, it also helps me step out of overwhelm when I'm feeling physically or emotionally drained. Ultimately, this pose makes me grateful for my body in any form.

Mindful Practice:

Knee-to-Chest Awareness

*From a seated position, ground down feet into the floor.

*Make sure your spine is long.

*Do a few rounds of breath to clear your mind and connect with inner awareness.

*On exhale, bring your left knee up and hold it with your hands and breathe in and out through your nose.

*If this movement strains your back, bring your knee up to where it feels good; you may try straightening your knee if that feels better in your body.

*We don't want to strain or push through pain. This is never our goal in the ancient practice of yoga or mindful movement.

*Always listen to the body, customize poses, and do what feels good to you.

*Try the other leg with breath.

*Repeat above mindful awareness a few more times, making sure to breathe with movement. Slow, deep awareness is our goal.

*When ready, answer the following prompt.

Exploratory Writing Prompt: When was the last time you practiced compassion for yourself and others? Describe the situation and how you felt. What opportunities or adventures do you want to create space for in your life? How do you see your life in 5, 10, or 15 years? What will you be doing, and where will you live?

Chapter 17
Mantra: I am powerful.

"I am incredibly, incredibly fortunate about the opportunities I've had. But at the same time, I've had plenty of opportunities to screw it up, too. Sometimes the most powerful thing you can say is 'No...' and not feel the need to do everything. It's about doing what rings true to me."

America Ferrera

I feel powerful when I make a choice. But as a former people pleaser, I realize I used to say yes to things even when I'd rather say no; I used to think I had to accept any opportunity that came my way. I rarely turned people down because I didn't want to cause friction. I wanted to avoid confrontation—I didn't want to hurt people's feelings. I also said yes because I was raised to think that you may miss out on things if you don't engage.

With age and maturity, I now realize that my belief was limiting. Now I know that I need time to sit with choices before deciding. I like to feel it in my bones, and when I feel relief, I know I'm on the right track.

When I say yes immediately—and don't take time to go within, tap into my inner wisdom, and feel my way through—I sometimes end up regretting decisions. I've learned that sitting with something and asking for guidance from God, or the Universe, and my inner wisdom always leads to better choices and living with ease.

In the end, making a choice from inner knowing leads to liberation because you know you have done what feels right for you. Use the following practice to step into your own power. Think of this pose as sweeping away doubt and ushering in power.

Mindful Practice:

Power Sweep

* Sit comfortably in your chair, elongate spine, look forward, and rest palms together in front of the chest at your heart center.
* On an inhale, sweep/raise up arms overhead, stretch hands upward, facing each other and apart with shoulders relaxed.
* On an exhale, hinge forward from hips, lower chest toward thighs to chair forward fold.
* Come down as far as comfortable for your body, round back, relax your head with arms hanging down, and sweeping behind you.
* You may stop at the floor if that feels good, or you may sweep your hands back behind you like a skier. Keep head relaxed.
* *Variation*: Put blocks in front to catch hands in forward fold instead of sweeping arms behind you.
* *Variation*: Move your hands underneath your knees with an elongated spine and flat back. Raise your head, neck, and chest, pressing your hands lightly below your knees if that feels good.
* Practice *Power Sweep* a few times with breath (in and out through your nose).
* Return to the center. When ready, answer the following prompt.

Exploratory Writing Prompt: Think back on a time when you said yes to something that you didn't want to do. How did this feel? Describe the emotions and sensations in your body. Did you feel numb, tense, queasy, heavy, or unstable? What choices can you make today to lean into your inner knowing?

Chapter 18
Mantra: I am open to new experiences.

"We proved that we are still a people capable of doing big things and tackling our biggest challenges."

Barack Obama

President Barack Obama fills me with hope and reminds me that we all have a responsibility to improve the collective good. No matter where we are in our healing journey, we have likely heard about the importance of reflection and developing self-awareness. For me, self-awareness is knowing my values and self-worth and knowing what is important to me. This includes knowing my thinking patterns and what motivates me, and my tendency to react to certain situations. It also includes my beliefs, principles, and dreams and what I hope to achieve or want out of life.

What obstacles do you face that keep you from living your dreams? If you could live the life of your dreams, what would it look like? These existential questions can mire us down, but when you grapple with them one by one, you begin to see that great things are possible if we tackle challenges one at a time. Living in the moment is our best defense at creating a world where everyone feels free.

The best thing we can do is enjoy every moment of our lives, and fully feel joy in every moment. One way I do this is by practicing *Open Arm Awareness*. Each movement expands my perception and opens my heart to possibility.

Mindful Practice:

Open Arm Awareness

*Ground down feet while sitting in your chair.

*Move towards the front of your chair. Or, if you have back issues, you may want to scoot back in the chair for support.

*Place hands on top of thighs, palms up. Wiggle fingers to release tension in your hands.

*Do several rounds of breath in this position (breath in and out through your nose), approximately 2-3 minutes.

*Then, on an inhale, stretch both arms wide to form a T. Imagine an invisible string-pulling your arms apart. Let up if you feel strain.

*Sit tall and elongate your spine. Continue nostril breath.

*Stay in this position for a few seconds…you can extend the time if that feels good to your body.

*On an exhale, release your arms and return your hands to the top of thighs, palms up, in receiving position.

*Do a few rounds of cleansing breaths as you return to your center.

**Variation*: You can also try moving one arm at a time in various positions. Feel free to explore. If this variation feels good, create a rhythm with your movement and nostril breath.

*If you embrace this pose early in the morning, it can wake up your entire body.

*When ready, answer the following prompt.

Exploratory Writing Prompt: Think of a situation where you acted on your beliefs. How did you come to know what was best? What physical signs told you to act upon your instincts? How did you feel? Describe the sensations in your body. Did you relax—did you feel quiet, secure, or safe? Name some of the physical signs that told you the next move.

Chapter 19
Mantra: Center. Breathe.

"Smile, breathe and go slowly."

Thich Nhat Hanh

Seamus Heaney once wrote, "I have begun to think of life as a series of ripples widening out from an original center." Finding and embracing my center has always been my goal in mindful practice. But I also love self-help books.

One of my favorites is *The Tools* by Phil Stutz and Barry Michels. This inspiring read offers helpful ideas on finding "courage, creativity, and willpower—and inspires [you] to live life in forward motion" (Stutz and Michels). The premise is that we all have a shadow self that keeps us from moving forward. But Stutz and Michels recommend that embracing our shadow can transform us.

For example, they say that by avoiding things, we set ourselves up for failure. That is, in the mere act of embracing and accepting what we fear, we can feel what we fear and create new, more productive outcomes. The more we learn to face fear, we change our perspective and reverse how we react.

My favorite chapter deals with confronting the comfort zone. Stutz and Michels say that we all want to avoid pain or avoid facing scary things, but the mere act of avoidance creates more pain. Therefore, most of us "barricade" into comfort to protect ourselves from feeling uncomfortable. The result: "[it] keeps our world small."

Keeping our world small may feel pleasurable and safe, but to take advantage of life, Stutz and Michels say, we must venture out: breaking through our comfort zone is the only way to step into and feel our full power.

The best way to do this is to carve out 5-10 minutes a day to center your mind and body with breath. I love the *Thread the Needle* pose because it relieves back pain but also stretches and expands my mind and body. Some practice this pose on the floor, but I prefer to practice in a chair. Feel free to play around with the hand and leg position. Either way, the following variation clears my head, makes me smile within, and reminds me to go slow and feel open to life.

Mindful Practice:

Seated Thread the Needle Variation

*Begin by sitting in a chair and grounding your feet into the floor.

*Sit tall with an elongated spine.

*On an inhale, lift your right leg and place your right ankle over your left leg, just above your left kneecap.

*Keep your left leg grounded—feel all four corners of your feet if you can.

*Do a full round of breath in and out through your nose.

*Then take left and right hands and clasp them together underneath your right leg. Left hand goes underneath your right leg and your right hand goes around outside of your right leg.

*Round your back slightly as you lean forward but listen to your body and avoid straining. For me, this pose relaxes my back and hips. But if you feel strain, opt out of arm movement, and place your hands on top of legs instead. Any mindful movement can be used. Feel free to explore.

*After a few rounds of breath in and out through your nose, switch legs.

*This practice can be done anywhere with a chair.

*Try this at your desk at work or at the airport.

*Enjoy!

*When ready, answer the following prompt.

Exploratory Writing Prompt: It is often said that a full life begins when we stop and smell the roses, but many of us have difficulty remembering this amid struggles. When was the first time in your life when you understood the importance of connecting with and becoming present in your life? If you don't have an example, write about how your connection with self could improve your world. Dive into this prompt with openness—add as much feeling and detailed description as you can. Try to see if there are places in your life to bring presence. State them here. Make a commitment to higher living.

Chapter 20
Mantra: I clearly see blessings all around me.

"It's never too late to become who you want to be. I hope you live a life that you're proud of, and if you find that you're not, I hope you have the strength to start over."

F. Scott Fitzgerald

If you're looking for simple ways to start over, find joy, and live by purpose, check out *The Happiness Project* by Gretchen Rubin. Rubin's fun, interactive book creates a yearly plan for living from happiness. Her book offers simple practices for maximum results.

Every decade in our lives offers new challenges. I truly believe we can reinvent ourselves as often as we like. This doesn't mean ignoring our true nature; it does mean we can step into our full potential if we trust that blessings are all around us.

When was the last time you thought about all the blessings of your life? Have you loved up on those who fill your cup, so to speak? Have you shared with loved ones and friends how much their presence in your life means to you?

Below is a practice that revives my desire for happiness. Mindfulness isn't a mysterious thing. In fact, the more you learn to reconnect with your inner world, the easier it becomes to benefit from taking a bite out of the happiness apple.

Rubin's book offers much insight on how to live self-actualized or become more self-aware. She talks about Benjamin Franklin's *Autobiography* and how he describes the "bold and arduous Project [of cultivating virtue]" in our lives. Rubin's book provides useful lessons for higher living. She also reminds us of the Buddhist saying, "When the student is ready, the teacher appears."

The following practice can rejuvenate the mind and body. Try this practice often, and you may feel a return in energy and vitality. You are your best teacher—listen to your inner wisdom. It can lead you to the life of your dreams.

Mindful Practice:

Vitality Reset

*Sit comfortably in your chair.

*Place your hands together at your heart center and rest them on your chest.

*Ground down feet and bring awareness to the body.

*Concentrate on your breath. Breathe in and out through your nose.

*How does this feel in your body?

*It might help to say to yourself: *my body feels open...I feel blessings all around.*

*Close your eyes and repeat this mantra.

*Now, continue to breath, and visualize a location that makes you feel a sense of well-being.

*Ask yourself: *Where am I? What are my surroundings? Describe the smell of the surroundings?*

*Now, once you have a vision or image, ask yourself: *what am I feeling in this space?*

*Use the breath to feel into the body and this moment.

*Let sensation wash over and cleanse your mind and body.

*Let go of all tension.

*Feel your body and mind, reclaim balance and vitality.

*Come back to this state for at least 2-5 minutes every day.

*Now, when ready, answer the following prompt.

Exploratory Writing Prompt: Think back to all the wonderful teachers in your life. Share anecdotes of the highlights, then dive into how these experiences or interactions improved your sense of self or helped form you into the person or the human you are today. These can be good or bad experiences. The point: tapping into previous experiences can help you discover what you learned from excellent teachers.

Accept

Section Five: *Accept*

Chapter 21
Mantra: Keep it simple.

"Life is really simple, but we insist on making it complicated."

Confucius

Most of our lives are filled with schedules and activities. I am most at peace when I keep things simple. But keeping things simple doesn't mean being lazy or passive. It means focusing our energy on what feeds us.

There is nothing simpler than placing your hands on a wall and becoming present in your mind and body. The following practice teaches inner awareness. As you learn to connect internally, mind and body expand, and you raise consciousness. Higher living can be a simple process. Self-acceptance can be yours if you keep going.

Mindful Practice:

Seated Wall Touch

*Turn your chair to face the wall.

*Sit in your chair with feet hip-width apart.

*Push your chair close to the wall but leave room for arm's length so you can stretch your hands to the wall.

*Let your arms relax and rest at the sides of the chair.

*Take a deep breath and relax your shoulders.

*Release tension throughout the body, now close your eyes.

*Take a few minutes to find a balanced breath in and out through your nose.

*On inhale, reach arms forward to touch palms on the wall.

*Lengthen your spine and breathe.

*Keep ears in line with arms—but if you feel strain, let up on your movement.

**Variation*: You may want to move your chair back and float your arms instead of pressing into the wall.

*Find the movement that suits your body.

*Root down or push down all four corners of your feet in the ground for support.

*Lift inner and outer arches down on the ground as you root palms into the wall or in front of you.

*Breath in this position for a few rounds of breath.

*Exhale as you release and return your hands to your heart center.

*Repeat the pose a few times.

*Try this pose anytime, anywhere.

*Return hands to your heart center and take a few cleansing breaths in and out through your nose.

*When ready, answer the following prompt.

Exploratory Writing Prompt: What can you let go of today? How are you holding on or building walls in your life? Are you pushing things away? How can you bring more awareness into your life and feel more like yourself?

Chapter 22
Mantra: Make friends with life.

"Look up at the stars and not down at your feet. Try to make sense of what you see and wonder about what makes the universe exist. Be curious."

Stephen Hawking

It took a lot of soul-searching to reclaim my life after my car accident. What I didn't know—or wasn't able to see or feel at the time of the accident—was that with every circumstance, health challenge, adversity, or hardship, God or the Universe was leading me to inner joy and a higher purpose. Pushing and striving toward external goals helped me survive for a while, but my soul knew there was a better way.

It's normal to feel negative when trauma occurs but left untreated, these feelings can dampen the human spirit. Old patterns can create walls for protection. I thought these walls protected me, but I was standing in my own way.

The truth is: we aren't put here to suffer; we're here to learn, adapt and grow. Trauma can trap us into making our lives small, but our challenges don't have to define us. My key to moving forward was making friends with life. Meditation, journal writing, and adaptive and accessible yoga unearthed whole-body acceptance. Inclusive, mindful practices brought liberation.

As mentioned before, by some miracle, I relearned to walk with foot orthotics but living in wholeness didn't happen overnight. My righteous anger and lack of self-compassion lessened over time and eventually pushed me toward sustainable healing.

In many ways, I've learned to redirect negativity into a more positive direction. I'm grateful for the many teachers and guides I've met on this journey. Each left wisdom and pushed me forward in unexpected ways.

Gradually I found the courage to own my body. It took years to learn that a strong will or ego doesn't always equal a strong mind and body. It took even more time to uncover a deeper understanding of myself and my health challenges.

Every experience, good or bad, has turned into a blessing. My car accident brought so much growth into my life. It taught me courage and willingness to embrace myself fully, flaws and all. Though challenging and unsettling, what once felt like torture now feels like a gift.

I love the simple act of placing legs up a wall. It's a wonderfully relaxing pose after a stressful day. It reduces edema and can relieve tension in the legs. I also like doing this pose before bed.

Mindful Practice:

Legs Up the Wall

*Lie on a bed or floor with feet against the wall.

*Move as close as you can so your bottom is against the wall.

*Relax your legs and feet as you take your legs up the wall.

*Release arms out to the sides, so they form a T shape.

*Lengthen the sides of the neck.

*Relax muscles in your face, throat, and tongue.

*Allow the weight of your legs to release into your hips.

*Feel your body let go of the tension of your day.

*Feel all your stress release as you passively allow the reverse the effect of gravity.

*This pose can also increase circulation in the lungs.

*Do deep breathing in and out through your nose, as you relax and release tension at the same time.

*When ready, answer the following prompt.

Exploratory Writing Prompt: Write about a challenging experience that turned into a blessing. If you're unable to think of one, write about a time when you faced adversity and how that experience changed you. What lessons were revealed?

Chapter 23
Mantra: I am here to flourish. I am blessed.

"I am not afraid of storms for I am learning how to sail my ship."

Louisa May Alcott

I was raised to believe we can make anything happen if we work hard enough and working hard brings fulfillment. Part of my work (teaching inclusive, mindful practices via YogiAble) is to teach others that adversity can make us stronger, but we can grow just as much, if not more, when we cultivate ease and joy in our lives. We don't have to fight the world or change ourselves to evolve. All we need is a desire to be authentic.

We can spend our lives searching for happiness outside ourselves, but everyone benefits when we share ourselves exactly as we are, raw and exposed. Humanity wins when we celebrate uniqueness.

In addition, I've found that my life flourishes when I embrace and accept all life's experiences. Corey Keyes defines this as flourishing. In general, Keyes says if we feel good but lack a higher purpose, we may find ourselves settling for less. On the other hand, Keyes also says if we are functioning well but lack happiness, we are striving, pushing too hard, and may feel unfulfilled.

The upshot: true transformation comes from within. I'm living proof you never know what life has in store. Big leaps are possible when we follow inner wisdom and trust what shows up. If we're bold enough to embrace fear and doubt, our life can unfold in incredible ways. We all can do this—we just need to trust ourselves.

While my journey continues to evolve, and I've just begun a new chapter publishing this book, I believe the world is working in our favor, and life experience brings us closer to a higher purpose. My journey has taken more than 40 years, but once I embraced vulnerability and claimed my authentic truth, I found gratitude and radical self-acceptance; everything became fuel for growth.

Therefore, I want to encourage people to stop searching outside themselves and cultivate acceptance within. I teach people how to explore, trust, and connect with their inner wisdom—this is where joy thrives—this is our birthright. We don't have to wait for difficulty to connect internally. It's available, portable, and free.

In the end, when we live in our flawed, whole being, and stand in our authentic truth, the path to wisdom is abundant. Learning to sail your own ship is possible if you stay true to yourself. The possibilities are endless.

Mindful Practice:

Inner Self Hug

*From a seated position and from hands at heart center, stretch arms out to either side in a "T" formation.

*Inhale and bring arms forward and around to give yourself a hug.

*Keep breathing as you observe the feeling of embracing yourself.

*What sensations come up?

*Enjoy this hug. This is your time—your practice.

*Keep breathing, inhale, and exhale as you hug yourself.

*Feel the nourishment.

*Rock gently from side to side - notice which arm is on top.

*Feel the rhythm of this pose in your body.

*Breathe.

*Release arms.

*Now, repeat *Inner Self Hug* with the other arm on top.

*Keep breathing in and out through your nose.

**Variation*: for a somatic approach, try tapping your hands one at a time while embracing yourself in *Inner Self Hug*.

*Release your arms back to center and take a cleansing breath.

*When ready, prepare to answer the following prompt.

Exploratory Writing Prompt: Are you sailing your own ship? That is, think back to a time in the last month when you did exactly what you needed for yourself. Write for 10 minutes on how that felt. Describe the feelings and sensations in your body. Did it lighten your load or increase your confidence? If so, how can you bring more of that into your life?

Chapter 24
Mantra: Dive into what scares you.

"The secret of change is to focus all of your energy, not on fighting the old, but on building the new."

Socrates

Learning to live with a spine injury wasn't easy. I felt traumatized, hopeless, angry, anxious, and sometimes I wallowed in my pain. I was 19 years old and didn't know how to handle my diagnosis. My physical challenges kept me fearful that I would never feel alive again. Some days my depression overwhelmed me. It took years to reframe my experience and understand that facing what scares us can lead to purpose.

My faith was the first step to healing, but I also did a lot of self-examination and research. At some point, I discovered Carol Dweck's Growth Mindset Theory, which deepened my awareness. Dweck explains how experiences (positive or negative) have the capacity to bring us deeper into our lives and embrace the truth of who we are.

More importantly, her work taught me that we don't have to push, strive, or work ourselves to death to find joy or happiness. We also don't have to hide our pain or rise above our circumstances to survive trauma. And even though our journeys may feel separate, our diverse stories are beautiful—our human flaws connect us. There is a treasure trove of gifts beneath our challenges; reframing this for myself opened my world.

Having a public online space, where I talk about my injury, and being visible on social media makes me feel vulnerable. But every time I share my story and my truth, I step into deep, personal growth. And guess what, I no longer want to deny my true self; I'm flawed and imperfect, but these are strengths, not weaknesses, and they need to be shared. I'm open to new challenges because they expand my reality and create possibility—that is the juice of life. Giving ourselves permission to fail and learning to recover with ease cultivates flourishing.

Mindful Practice:

Seated Forward Fold Awareness

* This pose can help stretch muscles in the back and thighs. It can also relax internal organs. Some say it can lower blood pressure.

* Begin by sitting in your chair.

* Press down evenly through sit bones.

* Extend both legs straight if this feels good.

* If not, I prefer to bend one leg at a time and ground four corners of one foot while keeping the other leg straight.

* Your choice.

* If you choose to bend one leg at a time, elongate your torso and over the center of your straight leg.

* On inhale, extend both sides of your waist evenly as you fold over your straight leg. Don't push or force your body down.

* Use your breath to feel into this action, breathe in and out through your nose (and rest over leg if that feels good).

* Keep fold centered, and don't overextend your straight leg.

*As always, listen to your body. We don't want to strain or push.

*Exhale as you return to beginning position.

*Now, try the other side.

*Use breath with action, while accepting your body in this moment.

*On exhale, release and bring your hands to heart center and take a couple rounds of slow, cleansing breaths.

*When ready, prepare to answer the following prompt.

Exploratory Writing Prompt: Having deep conversations with people can be scary. Experts say the mere act of confronting what scares us can bring us more joy and peace in our lives. Who do you need to thank in your life? Who do you need to set boundaries with? Who do you need to learn more from? Pick two of these questions and write for 5-10 minutes.

Chapter 25
Mantra: Accept who you are.

"Once we believe in ourselves, we can risk curiosity, wonder, spontaneous delight, or any experience that reveals the human spirit."

E. E. Cummings

I love this E.E. Cummings quote. It applies to so many things, including my adaptive yoga teaching and practice. Simply put, there are many yoga poses that don't fit my body. But I don't need to fret over this. Instead, I look for ways to adapt or customize poses for my body. Yoga and mindful practice can be accessible and inclusive for all bodies.

In addition, the beauty of mindful practice is finding and connecting with ease. It's not about competition or mastering poses. It's about self-acceptance, grounding, and expansion, and finding ways to accept who we are in the present moment. These universal truths are at the heart of my adaptive yoga practice.

The following practice brings calm to my body when I feel sluggish. If I practice this every day, I feel a deep inner connection to self-acceptance. Just like the E.E. Cummings quote, the more we believe in ourselves, the easier it becomes to risk curiosity and wonder. We can locate more joy in our experiences, which reveals the humanity or the human spirit.

I adapted the following pose to ease back pain. But if you have shoulder or arm pain, I'd pass on this pose. In my body, this feels like an inner connection and self-compassion. It's not about performance;

it's about feeling at home in my body. Any movement with breath is always a win.

Mindful Practice:

Seated Cow Face Variation

*Begin by sitting comfortably in your chair. Try moving to the front of the chair if this feels good. If not, sit in the back of your chair for support.

*Place hands on top of thighs in a receiving position.

*Take a few breaths in and out through your nose.

*Shift your weight in the chair so sit bones are evenly distributed on your chair.

*Cross your left ankle over your right ankle.

*Extend left arm to the ceiling with palm facing forward.

*Bend your arm at the elbow; you can rest your left hand on the top of your head if that feels good.

*Now, bring the right arm behind the back, rest on low back.

**Variation*: Since I sit back in a chair for back support, bring your right arm next to the right side of the chair, palm facing behind you if that feels good.

*You don't have to press or strain. Find what works for you.

*Take a few cleansing breaths in and out through your nose as you feel this action in your body.

*Reach through your fingertips and breathe.

*Move your right arm behind where it feels comfortable.

*Again, don't strain, push, or pull your arm.

*Rest your right hand on the back of your chair (instead of on your back) if that feels good.

*After a few rounds of breath with movement, return both arms back to your thighs with breath and end pose at heart center.

*Repeat the action by crossing your right ankle over your left, lifting your right arm up with your palm facing forward, and bending at your elbow.

*Then bring your left arm down the side of your chair and behind your back (if that feels good) with your palm facing down.

*Do several rounds with breath.

*Enjoy how this feels in your body.

*Release by returning to heart center in namaste or prayer hands.

*When ready, prepare to answer the following prompt.

Exploratory Writing Prompt: How can you practice more loving kindness and compassion for yourself? What can you do today to live more in balance and ease? Write down these reminders on note cards, sticky notes, or in your gratitude journal. The more you remind yourself of your inner power, the more you can live empowered.

Afterword

Now that you've read this book and applied the tools within, you may be wondering how you can come to every moment in your life with hope and possibility. How can you reframe disappointment for higher purpose? How can you live life as if you know the way? There is no one answer to these questions. In my experience, mindful practice is a practice. This path never ends. Therefore, I recommend starting your journey with a beginner's mindset. Every day is a fresh start.

When I first started mindful practice, I felt uneasy and self-conscious. I didn't know how to find stillness. I felt awkward, clumsy, and anxious. Overtime, I realized creating mindful practice is a non-linear choice. We all find time for many things in our day, why not create time for ourselves. Therefore, choosing one's own way is a choice and daily commitment.

When you choose to take care of yourself or find time to be still, you can reclaim balance, focus, cultivate more productivity and passion for life.

As you continue your journey, I want to leave you with two additional resources.

First, Viktor Frankl's life provides the perfect example of how making choices leads to freedom. In author Frankl's best-selling book, *Man's Search for Meaning*, he tells an inspirational story of what it was like to survive life in a concentration camp. Frankl's experiences demonstrate how he found hope despite suffering.

The truth is: we all have the capacity to learn and grow in our lives. We possess everything we need right now to find and live our own personal truth. It takes courage to step into our power.

Michael A. Singer's *The Untethered Soul: The Journey Beyond Yourself* is another helpful resource that has helped me on my mindfulness journey. In this delightful read, Singer says, "There is nothing more important to true growth than realizing that you are not the voice of the mind—you are the one who hears it."

In mindful practice, we do something similar—we observe our thoughts but don't judge what comes up; we merely remain open to possibility as our body moves and breathes. That's exactly what I hope for readers of this book.

True growth is a right of every human, but we're not raised to follow this path. Hopefully with the tools in this book, you can dive into the heart of what makes you tick.

Ultimately, I encourage you to explore the possibility of transformation.

For all of us, true, life-lasting growth is a lifelong journey. Growth is within reach when we trust ourselves.

I'm honored to welcome you to the party.

www.ingramcontent.com/pod-product-compliance
Lightning Source LLC
Chambersburg PA
CBHW041319110526
44591CB00021B/2838